Contents

D0255908

Perfect for holding back little mites...

New Allergy Control™ Perfect Covers are desig to encase your mattress, pillow or duvet, form a barrier to block the passage of housedust m and other allergens. Clinical studies have sho that this significantly reduces respirat symptoms in under 14 days. And unlike vinyl plastic covers, Allergy Control™ Perfect Cove allow water vapour to pass through easily, so y sleep comfortably.

So durable it's guaranteed for life...

The specially developed ACb2™ membrane Perfect Covers is so tough that we guarantee the for life. Our full range includes; Original Cove guaranteed for 20 years and Economy Cove guaranteed for 10 years.

IN USE AT THE LOW ALLERGEN HOUSE PROJEC
MILTON KEYNES

So inexpensive your savings can stay under the mattress!

This long working life allows for a regular vacuur or a damp wipe and hot washes at 60°C, an makes our Allergy Control™ Perfect Covers th most cost-effective allergy prevention system yo can buy.

Allerayde
Advancement in allergy protection

For further details complete the reply coupon and return to:
**Allerayde, FREEPOST (NG6287)
Newark, Notts. NG24 4BR**
Tel: 01636 613444 or Fax: 01636 611186

Please send me further information on:

☐ Perfect Covers ☐ Housedust mite avoidance

NAME
ADDRESS

POST CODE

☐ Our full range of environmental control products:

Allergy control vacuum cleaners and filters
Allergy control sprays and washes
Allergy control pillows, duvets and blankets
Room air cleaners and masks
Dust cloths, mildew and mould removers

Introduction

Hay fever, asthma, and other allergies have become much more common this century and are now important causes of illness, especially in children and young adults.

This booklet explains how allergies develop, describes the common symptoms, and gives detailed practical advice on how sufferers can recognise their own individual causes and avoid them.

It explains the medical treatments available, including self-help measures for emergencies.

Poor air quality from fuels has become very common this century There is no doubt that hay fever and asthma sufferers can be made worse on days of high pollution.

What is allergy?

Allergy is a word widely used to describe anything from an attack of sneezing and runny eyes on a warm sunny day, to an itchy red rash and wheezing after stroking the family pet, or to swelling of the lips and tongue and vomiting after eating a peanut. Allergy simply means an altered reaction, and is best thought of as the inappropriate and harmful response of the body's defence mechanism to substances which are normally harmless.

The commonest allergies are:

- hay fever and itchy eyes (allergic conjunctivitis)
- asthma
- itchy skin rashes
- food allergies
- allergy to wasp and bee stings.

Allergy to medicine and drugs such as antibiotics and local anaesthetics is less common.

Many asthma and hay fever sufferers find that taking aspirin and other similar drugs used to treat arthritis make their symptoms worse.

Many people who suffer a lot from stomach ache, diarrhoea and constipation, as well those experiencing severe headaches, hyperactivity or lassitude often put their problems down to food, although this is difficult to classify as true allergy; these reactions are best described as intolerances.

While you may get hay fever, asthma or itchy skin rashes (contact dermatitis) through breathing in or touching reactive chemicals at work, the environment in certain offices can cause what's known as 'sick building syndrome'. This is most likely in air-conditioned buildings which have artificial lighting, wall-to-wall carpet and windows that can't be opened. Symptoms include itchy eyes, dry throat and feelings of lassitude.

A number of people believe that they develop symptoms and feel unwell on contact with many of the chemicals used in everyday life, such as washing powders, bleaches, and aerosol cleaning sprays, and find it difficult to exist outside highly controlled environments free of such materials.

This is known as multiple chemical sensitivity and while it's real enough to the sufferers, it's difficult to explain scientifically and is at present not known to be a manifestation of allergy.

ALLERGY - A GROWING PROBLEM

There is no doubt that allergies are on the increase, although some are more common than others.

- One in three people will suffer from an allergy at some time in their life.
- One person in five suffers from hay fever. It was almost unknown until this century and like allergies in general appears to be a disease of prosperous countries.
- One in five schoolchildren is thought to be affected by asthma
- One in six children has skin conditions associated with allergy, particularly eczema.
- One in 20 people suffers the itchy raised rash known as urticaria.
- Food allergies, particularly to peanut, seem to be increasing at a dramatic rate though fortunately

they are still relatively uncommon, as is allergy to bee and wasp stings.

WHY IS ALLERGY MORE COMMON?

Allergies run in families. There are two key factors which determine whether you will develop an allergic disease. The first is your genetic make-up. The allergy gene controlling production of the allergy antibody, immunoglobulin E (IgE) and the inflammation that leads to allergic reactions, is positioned on chromosome 5. The second factor is your exposure to the allergen - the substance which causes the reaction. In most of the common allergies, you need to have encountered this early in life.

The rapid increase in allergies cannot be put down to a change in genetic make-up since this would take several generations, so it must be a result of changes in the environment and in lifestyle. An example of this process can be seen in the rapid increase in allergic diseases which is being detected in Eastern European countries that are rapidly assuming the Western European way of life. The kind of changes which are important include a decrease in worm infestation, fewer childhood infections and dramatic changes in living conditions in the home. The allergy mechanism is most effective at preventing worms in the gut

Heredity

Infections →

Passive smoking →

Cow's milk
other foreign proteins

← Dust mite

Pollutants →

Car exhausts ↗

↑ Exposure to allergens

Allergies can be triggered in genetically susceptible children if they are exposed to potential allergens in their first year of life.

entering the body. If this mechanism is no longer required to deal with worm infestation it is possible that it will now direct its effects against less harmful intruders such as pollen grains. Younger children in large families suffer much less from allergy than their older brothers and sisters. This is thought to be related to the more frequent viral infections readily passed from one child to another in large families. First-born children, in whom allergies are more common, escape these infections, which are thought to tilt the reactions of the immune system away from producing the allergy antibody. Smaller families mean a higher proportion of children affected by allergic diseases.

INDOOR AND OUTDOOR POLLUTION

Studies from Sweden, Germany and Japan have shown urban and rural differences in the frequency of the common allergic diseases. This suggests that modern-day pollution may be an important factor in the increase in allergic disorders. The most important components of this pollution are thought to be high levels of the oxides of nitrogen (NO_2) and, in particular, small particles present in the air in large numbers, largely due to emissions from diesel engines. Japanese and German studies have shown that allergies are more common in adults and children living within 100 metres of busy roads, compared to those living in less polluted parts of cities. These results have not been confirmed in the UK, possibly due to the fact that a major pollutant, ozone, can be found at high levels in the countryside, much of it being carried across from continental Europe. High levels of small particulates are also found in the air in rural communities. Although debate continues about the importance of air pollution increasing allergies, there is no doubt that those suffering from asthma and hay fever can be made worse on days of high pollution.

Indoor pollution is the major contributor to the epidemic of allergies seen today. The need to conserve energy, important as it is, has led to a transformation in the indoor condition in houses. Coal fires and lack of double glazing and insulation meant that houses in the past were draughty, with up to seven changes of the air in a room in every hour. Now that we have fewer chimneys, careful insulation, double-glazing and central heating, air exchanges in the rooms of modern houses may be less than one per hour.

As a result, humidity levels are high; most homes have more soft furnishings and fitted carpets, together creating an ideal environment for the house dust mite, and for the retention of allergens from pets, fumes from unventilated gas cookers, cigarette smoke and the fumes and vapours from household chemicals and sprays. This mixture of allergens and irritants in the unventilated home environment is likely to be the major cause of the rapid increase in allergic diseases.

WHAT CAUSES ALLERGY?

● The house dust mite, and particularly its droppings (faeces) is the commonest cause, affecting up to 90 per cent of allergy sufferers.

- Grass pollen causes a reaction in some 70 per cent of allergy sufferers, and the amount in the air will increase as more farmland is set aside for ungrazed meadows.

- Pets are the next most important cause of allergic symptoms with 40 per cent of asthmatic children sensitized to the allergens of cats or dogs.

- Trees are a common cause of early springtime hay fever. Global warming has meant that new plants, for example *Parietaria judaiica* or wall pellitory, previously confined to continental Europe, are now appearing in Southern England.

As warming increases birch pollen will become more of a problem, and even pollen from olive trees may be blown from Europe to the UK, as olive trees extend northwards from the Mediterranean.

- Moulds can trigger hay fever in the autumn, while spores from moulds such as *Aspergillus fumigatus* and *Alternaria* are very common in the atmosphere and can cause very severe attacks of asthma.

- Milk, egg, fish and now peanut are major causes of food allergy and colourings and preservatives can trigger attacks.

The droppings of the house dust mite, grass pollen, pets, tree pollen, moulds, milk, egg, fish and peanut are all common causes of allergy.

THE ALLERGIC REACTION

The allergic reaction begins early in life in people who are genetically predisposed. Exposure to both indoor and outdoor allergens, such as the house dust mite and pets, and pollens and moulds in a baby's first year leads to the production of the allergy antibody immunoglobulin E or IgE. The amount of exposure at this time is critical. A child who is exposed to high levels of house dust mite allergen in the home in the first year of life is statistically more likely to develop asthma in childhood and in the teens.

powerful chemicals called leukotrienes which can dilate blood vessels and constrict the smooth muscle encircling the airways of the lung. They also attract other specialized cells, particularly the white blood cells known as eosinophils, which can cause inflammation and damage.

Histamine and the leukotrienes cause itching and sneezing, together with swelling in the skin, in the tubes of the lungs (the airways of the lung) and in the lining of the nose, causing itchy red lumps in the skin, asthma, and nasal blockage. The inflammation in-

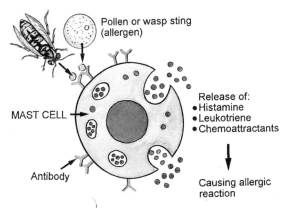

Contact with an allergen causes the mast cells to release histamine and other chemicals which cause allergic symptoms.

Similarly, children born during the pollen season are more likely to develop hay fever. IgE antibody fixes to specialized cells called mast cells which contain large amounts of histamine and other

duced by attraction of eosinophils leads to increased sensitivity of the lining of the nose and lung, and the development of chronic symptoms. Other cells, called lymphocytes, also play a key role in the persistent inflammation that characterizes eczema and contact dermatitis in particular but which is also a feature of hay fever and asthma.

How Allergy is Diagnosed

There are a number of possible tests which can detect whether your symptoms are due to an allergy and identify the allergen(s) responsible.

ulate what is happening in other parts of your body. A tiny prick is made into your skin with a needle or lancet through a drop of the allergen. Usually, the test will be done on the skin on your forearm or back. If the allergen provokes a release of histamine, you'll develop a red, itchy reaction within a few minutes. It then swells with a blister-like weal in the centre, reaching its maximum in about 20

The skin prick test can assess your reaction to up to 30 allergens at a time.

Skin prick testing

Mast cells to which the allergy antibody, IgE, has attached, are found throughout the skin and in the lining of the nose, the mouth, the tongue, the lung airways, and throughout the intestines. Your skin can be used as a test site to sim-

minutes and fading within a few hours. The size of the weal correlates roughly with the level of your allergy to that particular allergen. The prick test introduces such a tiny amount of allergen into the skin that testing is quite safe and can be carried out on almost any age group. Twenty to thirty allergens can be tested at the same time.

It takes some time for the mast cells throughout the body to become coated with IgE antibody and so skin tests may be negative in a child under the age of three, even though he or she is actually allergic to the allergen. Even when you have a positive test to a particular allergen, you may not get any symptoms when you come into contact with it because the body has mechanisms, at present ill-understood, which can dampen down the reaction to inhaled allergens. When positive skin tests correlate with symptoms, you can be certain that they are caused by an allergy to that particular allergen.

Skin patch tests

In this test solutions of common allergens causing contact dermatitis - such as ingredients of cosmetics, nickel or preservatives - are placed on the skin of your back and left under a special dressing for three days. If you develop an itchy, red raised patch, it means the result is positive. Taken in conjunction with a history of skin symptoms these tests have a high level of accuracy.

Blood tests

Blood tests (known as CAP-RAST) are increasingly used to test for the presence of IgE antibody in blood. Unlike skin tests they can accurately measure the precise amount of the allergy antibody in blood and the results are commonly graded on a scale of zero to six. When no or very little antibody (0 or 1) is found, you're unlikely to have any allergic disease, but moderate or high levels, (2 and above) are associated with allergic disease. As with skin testing, 20 or 30 allergens can be tested in one blood sample. These tests are particularly useful if you are taking an antihistamine which would block skin test reactions, or if you have widespread eczema, making skin testing difficult.

Other tests

A number of other tests for allergy are available. These include the neutralisation/provocation test (the Miller technique), cytotoxic tests of blood cells; hair analysis; Vega testing; applied Kinesiology and the auricular cardiac reflex method. The rationale for these tests is poorly understood and the results don't often match those produced by skin prick testing, patch testing or CAP-RAST testing. At the present time these tests are not recommended.

ANTI-ALLERGIC DRUGS

The most important factor in treating allergy is identifying the allergen which causes your symptoms, and avoiding contact with it as far as possible. However, there are several different groups of medicines which, when properly used, can not only relieve symptoms but also reduce the ongoing inflammation caused by chronic allergies.

Decongestants, broncho-dilators and emollients

- **Decongestant nasal drops or sprays** such as ephedrine and xylometazoline (Otrivine or Suda-fed) act by constricting the blood vessels supplying the lining of the nose, causing shrinking of nasal tissue and relief of nasal obstruction. These drugs act rapidly and are very effective, but you shouldn't use them for long periods at a time because shutting off the blood supply can cause tissue damage and worsening of your symptoms.

- **Bronchodilator drugs** work by relaxing the constricted smooth muscle which is narrowing the airways of the lungs of people with asthma. They act quickly and are very effective for people with mild asthma who only get occasional attacks of wheezing after contact with an allergen or after exercise. However, you shouldn't rely on them if your asthma is more severe since they do not treat the ongoing chronic inflammation. To stop this getting worse, you will also need treatment with inhaled anti-allergic drugs such as sodium cromoglycate (Intal) nedocromil sodium (Tilade) or steroids.

- **Emollients** soothe and moisturise the skin and are the basic treatment for all itchy, scaling skin disorders. Many different types are available, such as Aqueous cream, Diprobase and E45. Although there is little difference between them, you may find one suits you better than the others. Most people prefer to use creams which work into the skin rather than ointments which are greasy, and you may also be advised to add emollients to your bath water. Some people may develop an allergy to the preservatives contained in most emollients, however.

Other drug treatments

- **Antihistamines** were first discovered over 50 years ago and are the mainstay of allergy treatment. In the last decade several newer antihistamine preparations have become available, the so called 'second generation antihistamines'. These compounds such as terfenadine (Triludan), and cetirizine (Zirtek) have considerable advantages over the older 'first generation' antihistamines, such as chlorpheniramine (Piriton). Like the first generation antihistamines, they block the action of histamine released from mast cells and are very effective in the treatment of itching and sneezing. They have the advantage however of not crossing into the brain so they don't make you feel drowsy. This is a major plus point because it means that taking the drug doesn't interfere with your ability to carry out complex tasks such as driving or operating machinery. They are also less likely to make your mouth feel dry.

- **Anti-allergic drugs** - Intal and Tilade: This group of drugs remains unique in that they prevent the mast cells and eosinophils from releasing histamine and the other complex chemicals which cause inflammation. They have to be taken before you come into contact with the allergen - which means taking them regularly. Their remarkable lack of side-effects makes them very suitable for the treatment of allergic conditions, particularly allergic conjunctivitis, hay fever and asthma, especially in children who need long-term therapy when there is concern about the side-effects of other groups of drugs.

- **Corticosteroids** are powerful and effective anti-allergic and anti-inflammatory drugs. Although they do not block the release of histamine and other complex chemicals from mast cells, they are very effective at relieving the inflammation that characterizes chronic skin conditions associated with allergy, prolonged and severe hay fever (especially with a blocked nose) and moderately severe and chronic asthma. They operate at the level of the genes within the cells, preventing them from making important chemical messengers called cytokines, which influence the body's immune system at a very fundamental level.

While this group of compounds undoubtedly works well, there is concern about the side-effects which almost inevitably follow when you take any of them in tablet form. For this reason corticosteroids have been formulated as nasal sprays, for hay fever, inhalers for asthma, and creams for the treatment of skin allergies. In addition, the newer synthetic corticosteroids, such as budesonide (Pulmicort) and fluticasone propionate (Flixotide) are very effective on the surface of the lungs, nose or skin, but are not absorbed well into the blood stream. The small amount which is absorbed is rapidly removed again by the liver.

While we know that regular and prolonged use of steroid creams can lead to thinning and alterations in pigmentation of the skin, it is as yet not known fully whether the nasal and inhaled steroids have significant side-effects. There are concerns that the rate of growth in children may be reduced after prolonged and heavy usage of inhaled steroids. In addition, there have been instances of people bruising more easily and there is also the possibility that cataracts could develop in a person's eyes following use of these drugs. Corticosteroids remain the most effective treatment for allergies but they are most suitable for those people who have more severe disease which has not responded to other medicines.

Hay fever and itchy eyes

Attacks of sneezing, runny and blocked nose, together with itchy and watery eyes in summer was first called 'hay fever' in the middle of the 19th century. Although we still use the term, in fact fever is not a symptom of the disease, nor is it due to hay! A more accurate name is 'seasonal allergic rhinitis', the main cause of which is allergy to pollen. The symptoms of hay fever, or allergic rhinitis, can occur all year round, when it is called perennial rhinitis, and the main allergens involved are those from the house dust mite and pets.

Hay fever is the most common truly allergic condition and has become much more common in recent years, now affecting one in five of the population. As you'll know only too well if you're a sufferer, it's not just your nose that is affected. One of the most troublesome symptoms is itchy eyes that water all the time, a condition known as allergic conjunctivitis, and in up to a third of hay fever sufferers itching, red and running eyes are the major symptom. What's more, 50 per cent of hay fever sufferers also have symptoms of asthma. Hay fever is most common, and also at its most severe, in people in their teens, which causes particular problems because symptoms are at their worst in May, June and July - just when students have to take critical exams.

Sneezing and a runny nose can make life a misery for people with hay fever.

Eyes

Nasal passages

Ears

Throat

Your mouth, ears and throat can all be itchy when you have hay fever.

SYMPTOMS

Itching and sneezing

The most important job done by your nose is to filter air and protect your lungs. Itching and sneezing result from the effects of histamine released into the tissues of your nose during the allergic reaction to pollen. Irritation of just a very small area of the nose can result in instantaneous and vigorous sneezing, typically in bouts of five to 20 sneezes at a time. Your mouth may itch as well because pollen is swept from your nose into the back of your throat.

Some people find their ears itch too, not through pollen landing in their ears, but as the result of activation of a common nerve that links the back of the throat to the ear.

Runny nose

The nostrils are kept clear by secretion of a sticky fluid, mucus.

However, when you have an allergic reaction to pollen, your nose can secrete up to an egg-cupful of clean watery fluid every hour which spills out, so you're constantly sniffing and blowing your nose.

Stuffy, blocked nose

You may be among the half of all hay fever sufferers who have to put up with a blocked nose, the most distressing of nasal symptoms. This is the result of swelling of the nasal tissue caused by release of histamine and the leukotrienes from mast cells following interaction with pollen grains. When your nose is completely blocked, you suffer from headaches, disturbed sleep, mouth breathing and your throat and tongue feel dry when you wake up

Pollen grains can get into your eyes, making them itch and water. You rub them and then they itch and water even more.

in the morning. In severe cases, you can't smell or taste anything either.

Sinusitis

The sinuses, which are air-filled cavities in the bones of the skull, open out into the nasal cavity.

This membrane becomes inflamed making your eye look red, and you produce more tears to wash away the offending substance, causing your eyes to run. Particles accumulate in the inner corner of the eye,

Sinuses

Infected sinuses are very painful and make you feel quite ill.

When the tissue in your nose swells, it obstructs the openings and bacteria trapped in the sinuses multiply causing an infection. Acute sinusitis is very painful and leads to a fever and you feel really unwell.

Itchy, watering eyes

Pollen grains can easily get into your eyes, where they can react with mast cells present in the conjunctiva, the membrane which covers the white part of the eye and lines the inside of the eyelid.

which you then rub to remove them and this makes your eye itch all the more.

PERENNIAL ALLERGIC RHINITIS

This condition produces symptoms all year round. Although the major allergens are the house dust mite and pets, symptoms are often worse in the summer time due to additional allergy to pollen. A blocked, stuffy nose is a more frequent symptom of perennial compared to seasonal rhinitis, although allergic conjunctivitis is less common. Children with persistent year-round symptoms often have bags under their eyes. Many children wipe their noses with the palms of their hands, pushing the tip of the nose upwards and causing the development of a crease across the nose.

NASAL PRIMING

Most sufferers first develop symptoms of hay fever when the number of pollen grains in the air reaches 50 per cubic metre of air. However, as the season progresses and inflammation builds up, fewer and fewer pollen grains are needed to trigger an attack in the very sensitive linings of the nose and eyes. In addition, irritants in the air such as pollution and cigarette smoke, strong-smelling perfumes and household detergents and aerosols can also trigger attacks, making your life as a hayfever sufferer even

THE EFFECTS OF HAY FEVER

People who have never had hay fever tend to underestimate the symptoms you suffer as a consequence of this distressing allergy. A recent Gallup survey found that:

- Most importantly, 40 per cent of sufferers found that their work was affected by hay fever, mainly due to irritability and lack of concentration

- 80 per cent of sufferers felt really unhappy, miserable, depressed, irritated or listless during the hay fever season

- One in 10 said they had to take time away from work

- Studies have shown that children with hay fever perform less well in school

- 40 per cent of sufferers are self-conscious about the effects of hay fever on their appearance, causing restriction in their social lives

- 25 per cent of drivers who suffer from hay fever have said that their ability to drive was affected and that it was unsafe to drive when they had hay fever symptoms, which is obviously a significant finding more unpleasant. While you aren't actually allergic to these irritant substances, you are very sensitive to their irritating effects because the lining of your nose and eyes have become ultra-sensitive due to the continuing allergic reaction to pollen.

Many hay fever sufferers are allergic to the pollen from more than one type of grass.

THE ALLERGENS WHICH TRIGGER HAY FEVER

Hay fever sufferers are allergic to pollens present in the air. These come from wind-pollinated plants, by far the commonest of which are grasses, weeds and trees. Contrary to popular belief it is rare for suf-ferers to be allergic to pollens from brightly-coloured or scented plants, whose heavier, sticky pollens are transferred from plant to plant by insects.

Grass pollens

Amongst the hundreds of species of grasses only a relatively small number are sufficiently common and prolific pollen producers to give high atmospheric pollen counts. Rye grass, extensively planted for grazing, produces less pollen than the traditional meadow grasses, including Timothy grass, cocksfoot, Yorkshire fog, sweet vernal grass and orchard grass. As land is set aside from agricultural use, meadow grasses will once again dominate and as a consequence pollen counts are likely to rise.

There is extensive cross-react-ivity between the grass species, so if you're allergic to one type, you may react to some extent to others. The grass pollen season extends from mid-May to the end of July, peaking in late June and early July. The amount of pollen in the air varies from day to day and from hour to hour. Each grass species sheds its own pollen at a specific time of day. Although most species flower once daily in the early morning, two of the most prolific pollen producers, Yorkshire fog and sweet vernal grass, flower for a second time in the late afternoon.

Magnified poliens (left to right): Timothy grass, Scots pine and Golden rod.

Tree pollens

The major sources of tree pollens are hazel, plane, oak, elm, ash and birch, and the pollen is produced in the spring shortly after the leaves develop. The tree pollen season is shorter than that of grass pollen, lasting between four and six weeks from the end of March to the beginning of May.

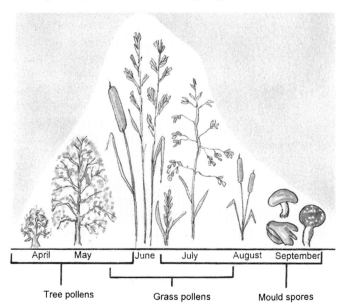

| April | May | June | July | August | September |

Tree pollens   Grass pollens   Mould spores

Different allergens predominate in the air according to the time of year.

Hazel

London Plane

Warty Birch

Tree pollen appears soon after the leaves open in early spring.

Weed pollens

Unlike North America and the Mediterranean coastline, the climate of the UK does not favour the growth of ragweed, which is one of the most prolific pollen producers. Stinging nettle leaves are covered with hairs which inject histamine-releasing factors into the skin,

causing the typical pain, itching and rash. Nettles flower in late summer and autumn, injecting pollen into the air as the sun shines on the curled young flowers. Fortunately, allergy to their pollens appears relatively uncommon. However a member of the same family, *Parietaria judaiica*, better known as wall pellitory, produces large amounts of highly allergenic pollen, and is a major cause of hay fever symptoms in continental Europe. However, this plant has gained a foothold in southern England where it has begun to cause symptoms in late summer and early autumn.

Brassica napus -oil seed rape

The last decade has seen a great increase in the cultivation of this plant. Pollination is part by wind, and part by insect. Although the bright yellow colour of the flower makes its presence obvious, few people are truly allergic to its pollen.

Moulds

Moulds, a sub-division of the fungi, are very adaptable and may be found anywhere where there is moisture and oxygen. Typically they consist of long filaments which grow on the surface of organic materials such as compost heaps or rotten fruit or cheese.

Cladosporium herbarum: This mould produces a very large number of spores and is the most commonly encountered mould allergen. Particularly heavy concentrations occur between May and October, reaching up to 15,000 spores per cubic metre of air. The wood, and is a major cause of allergic disease in the USA. In this country *Alternaria* causes rhinitis and asthma in the autumn, particularly during harvest time.

Microscopic spores from moulds, which are a type of fungus, appear in late summer and early autumn.

mould colonizes foliage and plant matter, particularly grass, and the spores are a cause of hay fever during the summer months, particularly when the grass is mown. Allergy to *Cladosporium* may be why your symptoms do not coincide with the grass pollen count.

Alternaria alternata: This is another extremely common mould, found in soil compost and rotten

GLOBAL WARMING

Some temperate areas of Europe, including southern England, have shown an increase in temperature of up to 0.5 degrees Centigrade since 1970. If this trend continues life will be even more unpleasant for hay fever sufferers. The hay fever season would extend with grasses flowering earlier in the year and continuing into the late autumn. In addition birch pollen would be produced earlier in the year and some people could develop allergy to pollen from olive trees. Most worrying is the possibility that ragweed could establish itself in the UK. The pollen is potent, with fewer grains needed to produce attacks of hay fever. Ragweed is a prolific producer of pollens, leading to the severe hay fever experienced by sufferers in the USA.

WEATHER AND THE TIME OF DAY

Grass flowers open early in the morning and pollen is scattered into the air. On fine, clear days, as the temperature rises, air carries the pollen up through the atmosphere, sometimes to the height of cumulus clouds. When these convection currents cease as the Earth's surface cools in the early evening, pollen grains fall in concentrated clouds. The peak concentration of pollen in country areas is around 5.00 - 6.00 pm, while in urban areas the peak is delayed by one to two hours. On calm nights, pollen from high in the atmosphere will gently settle out in the still air, resulting in a second peak after midnight. This pattern can be disrupted by rain in the morning, delaying the opening of the grass flowers and, if it persists, reducing pollen counts that day.

Daily estimates of the pollen counts expressed as the average number of grains per cubic metre of air during a 24 hourperiod, are regularly reported during the spring and summer in newspapers and on television and radio weather broadcasts.

Thunderstorms can have a dramatic effect on the level of pollen allergen in the air. This is due to the fact that the high humidity prior to the storm causes pollen grains to burst, liberating hundreds of small starch particles which carry one of the major grass allergens. In cities the allergens can attach to small carbon particles in the air, themselves the product of diesel engines. The starch granules, or allergens, combined to carbon particulates are readily inhaled, not only into the nose, but also into the airways of the lung, and were the cause of the remarkable outbreak of asthma in June 1994, which led to a dramatic increase in hospital admissions among hay fever sufferers who had never previously suffered from asthma. In addition, thunderstorms can lead to a dramatic increase in spore counts from a mould called *Didymella exitalis*, which is found on the leaves of ripening barley and wheat. The release of spores increases 25-fold after the start of the rainfall.

TREATMENT

The treatment for hay fever, as with other allergies, is based on avoiding the allergen. Since clouds of pollen grains are blown into urban areas counts can be high, even in the centre of large cities, and you can't avoid them altogether. However there are some steps you can take to reduce your exposure to pollen.

- Avoid being outdoors in the early evening when pollen counts are at their highest
- Be aware of the pollen count and try to stay indoors when it is high
- Sleep with your bedroom windows closed to prevent pollen entering on still, calm nights
- Wear sunglasses which can help to prevent pollen getting into your eyes
- Get someone else to mow the lawn
- When you're in the car, keep windows and doors closed; when buying a new car choose one with a pollen filter in the ventilation system
- Take your holidays in coastal areas where sea breezes keep pollen inland
- Take a shower and wash your hair when coming indoors in the evening to get rid of pollens.

FOOD ALLERGY

Food allergy rarely causes hay fever-like symptoms. However, some people find that cutting out dairy products from their diet alleviates nasal symptoms to some degree, particularly excessive nasal secre-tions. There is cross-reactivity between birch pollen and certain fruit allergens, particularly apples. About one in 20 people who have perennial rhinitis are sensitive to aspirin and other non-steroidal anti-inflammatory drugs such as ibuprofen (Nurofen), which can trigger symptoms and are associated with the development of nasal polyps.

MEDICINES FOR HAY FEVER

The management of hay fever has been transformed by the fact that you can now buy virtually all the necessary treatments over the counter from the pharmacy without a prescription.

Decongestants

Oxymetazoline (Afrazine) and xylometazoline (Otrivine) as nasal drops or sprays are the most commonly used decongestants. They act rapidly and help clear your blocked nose quickly and effectively. Their effect lasts for a relatively short time when they're used in this way. Ephedrine nasal drops are an alternative. Topical decongestants also work very well, but you have to remember not to go on using them for more than 14 days. Using them for long periods can cause damage to the lining of the nose, making the blocked nose worse than ever once the effect of the drug has worn off. As a result, you're tempted to use them more

The British Allergy Foundation has developed a series of goals for the management of hay fever. These are:

1 The ideal is to allow sufferers to be free of the limitations caused by hay fever so that they can carry on with work or school as usual and enjoy the spring and summer.

2 Treatment should be aimed at reducing all symptoms of hay fever, including sneezing, runny nose and eyes, and nasal blockage.

3 In moderate and severe cases treatment should be aimed at the underlying inflammation.

4 Side-effects of treatment should not interfere with, or restrict, sufferers' daily activities or quality of life.

5 Hay fever treatment should not prevent the sufferer from being able to drive or operate machinery.

6 In order for sufferers to comply with therapy, dosage should be simple.

7 There should be minimal risks of side-effects.

8 There should be no interactions with other medication the sufferer is taking.

and more often to try and clear your nose. Decongestants are particularly useful in relieving nasal blockage before using an anti-inflammatory drug.

Antihistamines

As you can now buy the modern, non-sedating, second generation antihistamines from the pharmacy, you should always opt for one of these instead of the older, sedating, antihistamines such as chlorpheniramine (Piriton), or clemastine (Tavegil).

Although these antihistamines are rarely associated with any drowsiness, you should take care when driving and avoid drinking too much alcohol. Astemizole and terfenadine have been associated with the development of serious rhythm disturbances of the heart in a very small proportion of hay fever sufferers. This is particularly the case in people taking the anti-fungal drug ketoconazole or the antibiotic erythromycin at the same time. Since there is little to choose between the effectiveness of these

CHOOSING THE RIGHT ANTIHISTAMINE

These are all non-sedating, newer antihistamines which you can buy from the pharmacy without a prescription.

Generic name	Brand Name	Daily Dose
Cetirizine	Zirtek	10 mg once in the morning
Loratadine	Clarityn	10 mg once in the morning
Astemizole	Hismanal	10 mg once in the morning
Terfenadine	Triludan	60 mg twice daily

These antihistamines can be sold for the treatment of hay fever in children over the age of 12, and in the case of Triludan, for children over the age of six. Your doctor can, however, prescribe these antihistamines for younger children. Loratadine can be prescribed for children over the age of two.

drugs it's best to avoid those associated with side-effects if possible. On this basis loratidine and cetirizine can be recommended as the first choice antihistamines.

Not everyone responds to the same extent to each of the antihistamines and you may need to try one or two before finding the preparation that suits you best.

There is another antihistamine called acrivastine (Semprex) which is only available at the moment from your doctor. This needs to be taken three times a day.

Antihistamines can be sprayed directly into the nostrils, and one preparation, azelastine (Rhinolast) is available as a twice daily nasal spray. Whilst this preparation is very effective for the nasal symptoms of rhinitis, it does not, unlike the antihistamines taken by mouth, have any effects on allergy symptoms affecting the eyes.

Anti-allergic preparations

These are the mainstay of treatment for more persistent rhinitis and need to be taken on a regular basis.

STEROID NASAL SPRAYS

Generic Name	Brand Name	Dose	Available direct from a pharmacy?
Beclomethasone dipropionate	Beconase Hayfever	2 sprays to each nostril morning and evening	Yes
Flunisolide	Syntaris	(ditto)	Yes
Budesonide	Rhinocort	(ditto)	No
Fluticasone propionate	Flixonase	2 sprays to each nostril once daily in the morning	No

While all these preparations are very effective, Fluticasone (Flixonase) is probably the safest and most potent medicine for the treatment of hay fever but it can only be obtained on prescription from your doctor.

Sodium cromoglycate (Rhinacrom) prevents allergen interaction with the mast cell from releasing histamine and the leukotrienes which is what causes your symptoms. It is useful in persistent rhinitis in both adults and children, and as a four per cent aqueous spray can be used between two and four times a day.

You can buy it over the counter from the pharmacy in the form of Resiston 1, which is a combination of 2 per cent sodium cromoglycate spray together with xylometazoline as a decongestant. Sodium cromoglycate is much more effective in treating allergic conjunctivitis where it can be applied as eye drops up to four times a day, or as an ointment to treat itchy eyelids. You can buy them from the pharmacy without a prescription as Clariteyes or Opticrom. These eye drops contain a preservative called benzalkonium which can itself occasionally cause an allergic-type reaction. When you're using these eyedrops or ointment, you shouldn't wear soft contact lenses as they could react with the preservative.

Corticosteroids

These are the most effective treatment for moderate and severe hay fever, particularly when symptoms are persistent and include nasal blockage. They reduce inflammation in the lining of the nose and treat all symptoms effectively. For reasons that are not wholly understood spraying these medicines into the nose also helps to relieve allergic conjunctivitis. The nasal sprays should be used regularly on a daily basis.

Corticosteroids can be given as tablets which act rapidly and very effectively and can be used over a period of up to 14 days. They give you complete freedom from symptoms and are ideal for specific periods when you need to be on top form - for example, for key examinations or a wedding. Long-lasting injections of corticosteroids are not recommended because of side-effects.

Hyposensitization (specific allergen injection immuno-therapy)

This type of treatment involves injecting increasing amounts of purified grass pollen solution under your skin until your sensitivity to the allergen is reduced. To get the full benefit, you need to have injections monthly at the maximum dose over a period of two to three years.

This treatment can be very effective in severe hay fever which has not responded to anti-inflammatory treatment. Because of the dangers of severe reactions which can include collapse (anaphylaxis), the injections can only be given in specialist hospital clinics where full resuscitation facilities are available. Those undergoing this treatment must be carefully observed for 60 minutes after each injection.

Asthma, cough and wheezing

A sthma is the only chronic disease in the developed world which is becoming more common. Studies of school children have shown that there has been a fourfold increase in the numbers suffering from asthma over the last 20 years. Asthma is now the commonest reason for children to be admitted to hospital and in many areas is one of the leading causes of hospital admissions for adults as well. Tragically asthma kills over 2,000 sufferers per year, many of them under the age of 35. Allergy is the most important cause of asthma, being implicated in 90 per cent of children and 50 per cent of adults with the disease.

WHAT IS ASTHMA?

The word asthma derives from Greek and literally means hard breathing, but its modern definition includes a description of its symptoms, the underlying mecha-

nisms causing the disease, and its effect on the function and sensitivity of the lungs and their airways.

Normal airway

Airway in spasm

During an asthma attack, the airway becomes constricted, making it difficult to breathe.

The symptoms of asthma are coughing, wheezing and shortness of breath, but the condition is characterized by a special type of inflammation of the lining of the airways of the lung. The key cells involved, as in other allergic diseases, are the mast cell and the eosinophil.

The effect of this inflammation on the lungs is to cause narrowing of the airways with a reduction in the amount of air that can be blown out of the lungs in a given time, and in the rate at which air can be expelled from the lungs. This obstruction to the flow of air out of the lungs can be completely or partly reversed by the inhalation of a bronchodilator. In addition, the inflammation of the airways causes them to be hypersensitive to many irritants such that the inhalation of cold air, pollution fumes, aerosols, household cleaning agents and disinfectants and strong scents can trigger constriction of the irritated airways, giving rise to attacks of asthma.

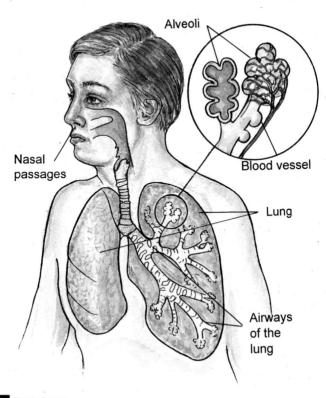

Alveoli

Nasal passages

Blood vessel

Lung

Airways of the lung

SYMPTOMS

Shortness of breath

Difficulty with breathing, a feeling of tightness in the chest, and shortness of breath are the cardinal features of asthma. Their severity can vary from a short-lived feeling of breathlessness after exercise or after stroking the family pet, to disabling breathlessness, such that you cannot walk and don't have enough breath to complete a sentence. The hallmark of asthma is the variability in symptoms, so that on some days you feel fairly well, while at other times you may need urgent treatment.

Wheezing

This whistling sound is the result of air being forced through swollen and partially obstructed airways in your lungs, causing whistling noises of different pitch. Wheezy breathing is easily recognised but it may not happen when the asthma is severe because insufficient air is being blown out through the airways of the lungs to generate the noise.

Coughing

A cough, especially at night, is a characteristic of asthma, as it is of many other lung diseases, particularly bronchitis induced by smoking or associated with a chest infection. It can be difficult for a doctor to diagnose whether a cough is actually the result of asthma rather than of some other lung condition. Inflammation of the lung airways in babies and toddlers is frequently the result of viral infections. Infection with the respiratory syncytial virus gives rise to a troublesome and sometimes serious condition called bronchiolitis, which makes the lung airways (the bronchi) swell up. The young child suffers wheezing and breathlessness as well as fever. He or she will often have a cough for some time after one of these viral infections and if there is a family history of asthma, this may be the first sign that the child is developing it. It is not surprising that young children are often treated with frequent courses of antibiotics before the correct diagnosis of asthma is made and appropriate treatment with bronchodilators, anti-allergic and anti-inflammatory drugs started. Similarly it can be very difficult to distinguish between bronchitis and asthma, particularly in adults who smoke and who are suffering prolonged episodes of coughing. It is important to make the correct diagnosis since bronchitis must be treated with antibiotics, while, on the other hand, an asthmatic cough will respond to appropriate anti-asthma treatment. Either way, it's important to stop smoking.

Night-time

All the symptoms of asthma worsen during the night, disturbing your sleep and leaving you feeling tired next day. The reason for this is that lung function in everybody is at its worst at four in the morning and at its best at four in the afternoon. This is due to the changes that occur in circulating levels of the hormone adrenaline which are lowest in the middle of the night. Adrenaline helps to relax the muscles of the lung airways keeping them open. As the body shuts down during sleep nerve impulses slow the heart and the activity of the intestines, but at the same time cause minor narrowing of the airways of the lung. In addition circulating levels of corticosteroids, so important in countering any inflammatory process in the body, are low in the early hours of the morning. While you won't ever notice these effects if you don't have asthma, their influence is greatly exaggerated in people who already have inflammation of the lung airways, making their symptoms and lung function worse at night.

Exercise

Inhaling cold dry air by breathing through your mouth when you're exercising leads to changes in the fluid lining the lung airways, triggering off release of histamine and other potent chemicals, including the leukotrienes, from mast cells. This leads to a brief attack of asthma lasting 10-20 minutes and can have a devastating effect on a child's ability to join in games in the playground and on the playing field, disrupting social and physical development.

GETTING THE RIGHT DIAGNOSIS

In order to decide whether you have asthma, the doctors need to find out whether the degree of obstruction to the flow of air through your lung airways varies at different times. This task has been made much easier with the introduction of small airflow meters which you can use yourself to record the maximum rate at which you can blow air out of your lungs at different times of the day. The most widely used meter, available on prescription, is the Wright mini peak flow meter. You blow as hard as possible through the meter and record the peak expiratory flow rate (PEFR). The maximum PEFR depends on your age, sex and height, and various from approximately 600 litres per minute in a fit young man of average height to approximately 300 litres per minute in an older woman. Recordings in people with asthma show a reduced peak flow measured when they wake up compared to peak flows measured in the early evening. This pattern of variation is the same each day. A variation in the peak flow from morning to evening of 15 per cent or more confirms the diagnosis of asthma.

The peak flow meter is also useful in monitoring the effects of treatment, which reduce the variation as well as improving the peak expiratory flow rate overall, since the more severe the asthma the lower the PEFR.

More sophisticated tests can be undertaken in special hospital lung function laboratories. These include the measurement of the amount of air that can be blown out of the lungs in one second (the forced expiratory volume in one second, or FEV1). This is an accurate test because the amount is reduced in asthma sufferers. An improvement in the FEV1 of 15 per cent or more after the inhalation of a bronchodilator confirms the diagnosis of asthma. Exercise or inhalation of solutions of histamine can be used to stress the lung, inducing a brief, short-lived fall in lung function in people with asthma.

IDENTIFYING THE ALLERGENS
The house dust mite

The house dust mite, or to give it its proper name, *Dermatophagoides pteronnysinus* (from the Greek meaning skin eating feather mite), is the source of the major allergen causing asthma in the UK. It is one of almost 50 species of mites and has adapted very successfully to life in our homes. It is essentially a bed mite, since it feeds on human skin scales which are shed into our bedding during sleep. There is no shortage of food since one person sheds 0.5 - 1 gram of scales each day, sufficient to feed thousands of mites for months. Since their diet of skin scales is essentially dry, mites need to obtain fluid from the air and for this reason the humidity in the atmosphere is usually the decisive factor determining the size of the mite population. Conditions of approximately 80 per cent relative humidity and 25° Centigrade of warmth form an ideal habitat for mites. In London the average monthly humidity varies between about 73 per cent in June to about 86 per cent in December, and it's not surprising that levels of infestation in British homes are high. In mountainous areas, particularly above 1400 metres, mites are found in very low numbers, probably as the result of the low humidity at altitude and low temperatures. Mites vary in numbers in

The droppings of the house dust mite are the major cause of allergic asthma.

dust collected from mattresses but infestation can be as high as 5000 mites per gram of dust.

The mites themselves are very small, approximately 0.3 mm in size, and are indistinguishable from specks of dust to the naked eye. Under the microscope they look pretty unprepossessing. Despite their small size intact house dust mites are far too large to inhale deep into the nose or lungs and studies have shown that the allergen causing asthma is found in the droppings or faeces of the mite. The allergen itself is a protein excreted by the mite's gut that is used to digest the human skin scales that it has eaten. These faecal pellets are approximately 20 microns in size, that is, 20,000ths of a millimetre. They can easily be breathed into the nose, where they cause perennial rhinitis, and fragments are easily inhaled into the lungs where they cause the allergic reaction that leads to asthma. The chemical nature of the house dust mite allergen has been fully worked out and is called Der p1.

Apart from the bedroom they're found in greatest numbers in living rooms. Carpets and upholstered furniture can develop high mite counts in excess of 1,000 mites per gram of dust and extremely high levels of the mite allergen. You inhale mite allergens when dusting or vacuuming, and during the night from bedding as you continually move around while sleeping. During his or her first year of life, a baby who is born with an inherited predisposition to allergy can become sensitized to the house dust mite if exposed to 100 mites per gram of dust from mattresses and carpets. Severe attacks can be triggered at levels of 500 mites per gram of dust.

Pets

Pets are now one of the major causes of allergic disease, second only to the house dust mite, with up to 40 per cent of asthmatic children sensitized to the allergens of cats and/or dogs. It is not necessary to be in direct contact with a cat or dog for an attack of asthma to occur. Animal allergens are present in the air and dust in the home, and allergy sufferers can develop asthma as soon as they go into a home with a pet. The allergens themselves are found in dander (skin scales), hair, saliva and urine, and get everywhere in the home where the animal lives. Cat allergens are found mainly in the saliva, the sweat ducts and the tear ducts. The fur becomes coated with the allergen during grooming. Cat fur itself is not intrinsically allergenic. A cat can shed 0.2 grams of hair and dander each day, leading to high concentrations of this potent allergen in the house.

Dog allergen in the home comes mainly from dander, hair and saliva. Quite often an asthma sufferer will have problems with some breeds but not others. There is some suggestion that the offending allergen is the same in all breeds, and it is just the concentration which varies.

Rabbits, small rodents and caged birds are very popular pets. Rabbits and guinea pigs are usually housed outdoors, whereas gerbils, hamsters, mice, rats and birds are more likely to be kept in the living room or even in the bedroom. These creatures, especially budgies and hamsters, are particularly associated with allergic asthma. In small mammals, urine is the most potent source of allergen, and materials lining cages can be heavily contaminated. Allergens are released into the air as the animal moves round the cage, disturbing the lining.

Moulds

Apart from *Alternaria*, which can cause asthma in the autumn, the spores from *Aspergillus fumigatus* are an important cause of severe asthma. *Aspergillus fumigatus* is widely distributed, and found particularly in rotting vegetation.

Occupational allergens

Reactive chemicals and allergens encountered in the workplace are

Cat

Dog

Hamster

Family pets, especially cats, dogs and hamsters, are a major cause of allergic disease in children.

10 STEPS TO PREVENTION

1. Reduce moisture and damp. Open a window or door to ventilate your bathroom and kitchen during and immediately after cooking, washing and bathing. To avoid moisture spreading to the rest of the house keep the internal doors closed. Don't dry clothes indoors unless dryers are vented to the outside. Air bedding before making beds and maintain a background ventilation in bedrooms by keeping a window open whenever possible.

2. Prevent build-up of dust. Reduce the number of exposed surfaces on which dust builds up, especially if they are difficult to clean. Clean surfaces with a damp cloth. Vacuum clean soft furnishings and curtains, as well as carpets and floors with a properly maintained cleaner. Vacuum clean mattresses fortnightly. Replace pillows and buy new ones every three months if you can.

3. Wash bed linen at a high temperature (at least 60° Centigrade) to kill the house dust mite.

4. Enclose bedding and wash soft toys. Encase all mattresses, duvets and pillows in the sufferer's bedroom with microporous membrane covers. Many different types are now available and the costs vary. These covers need to be wiped clean with a damp cloth and completely dried each time you change the bed. Soft toys can contain large numbers of house dust mites, so choose ones that can be washed at 60° and other toys that can be wiped down and keep soft toys out of your child's bed.

5. Get rid of carpets. Wherever possible replace them with linoleum or vinyl flooring, or sealed natural flooring such as cork tiles or wood, with as few dust-retaining crevices as possible.

6. When replacing your vacuum cleaner, choose one of the high efficiency filter models - look for the Allergy Friendly logo of the British Allergy Foundation.

   allergy / friendly
   british allergy foundation

7. Replace furnishings. Get rid of woven fabric-covered chairs or sofas and opt instead for cane, canvas, leather or leather-like covered furnishings which are easy to clean and do not harbour house dust mites.

8. Changing your home environment: although not yet proven it is likely that a different type of heating system with improved through drafts will reduce humidity and house dust mite numbers. Air filtration,

dehumidifiers and mechanical ventilation with heat recovery are all being tried. The National Asthma Campaign, working with a building company, have created the first low allergen house which embodies these steps to reduce exposure to allergens. This approach is a step in the right direction for the millions of sufferers of house dust mite allergy.

9 If at all possible, find a new home for your cat and/or dog. Perhaps surprisingly, giving your pet frequent baths can be effective. Bathing a cat once a week can reduce the allergens in the home by 90 per cent, although the cat may not like it much. Unfortunately confining a cat to one part of the house is unlikely to be effective as people transfer cat allergens to other parts of the home on their clothes as they move from room to room. Sadly, in allergic families, pets need to be banned. Even after the animal has gone it can be many months before the allergen levels in the dust fall, and allergens can only eliminated completely by replacement of all floor coverings and upholstery, and by thorough cleaning.

10 Reducing humidity and dampness in your home will effectively prevent the growth of the moulds that can cause asthma and other allergies. Awareness and recognition of occupational causes of asthma can lead to effective industrial hygiene, eliminating the problem altogether.

an important cause of asthma, particularly in adults who also smoke. It's very important to recognise the possibility that dusts, vapours or fumes which you encounter at work may be the cause of your asthma, since avoiding the sensitizing agent may get rid of it completely. On the other hand, if you are constantly exposed to the allergen over a long period of time, your symptoms may persist and even become permanent.

The commonest cause of occupational asthma is contact with the chemical toluene diisocyanate used in varnishes and paints. Soldering fluxes in the electronics industry and platinum salts encountered in metal refining are also important causes. Bakers can become allergic to flour and farmers and dock workers allergic to grain, and indeed to the grain mite that flourishes in grain with a high water content. Carpenters and sawmill workers can become allergic to dusts from wood, and those working in the pharmaceutical industry to a number of the medicines manufactured. Increased recognition of this problem and considerable improvements in ventilation and hygiene should reduce the number of sufferers from occupational asthma.

The characteristic feature, which tends to confirm the diagnosis of occupational asthma, is that symptoms occur soon after starting the working day, but improve at weekends and may disappear on holidays.

TREATMENT

At the present time there are no medicines which can cure asthma. For this reason it is essential to try to minimise exposure to the important allergens that can initially sensitize babies in the first year of life, and subsequently cause attacks of asthma. This can be done in a step-wise approach (page 38).

AIR POLLUTION

There is no doubt many people suffer attacks of breathlessness and coughing - whether they have asthma or not - during episodes of air pollution caused by emissions from petrol and diesel engines and from the burning of coal and gas in power stations. When you do have asthma, the effects of pollution reduce the amount of allergen needed to bring on an attack. What's more, pollution may bring on attacks of asthma in people who had previously only suffered from allergic rhinitis. The cocktail of pollutant gases, sulphur dioxide, ozone and the oxides of nitrogen, together with small particulates, less than 10 microns in diameter, emitted from diesel engines (PM10's) may be particularly dangerous and lead directly to the death of people with severe asthma and other respiratory diseases. Whether pollutant gases are an important contributing factor to the increase in asthma remains to be determined.

Other triggers

Viral infections, particularly with the common cold virus (known as the rhinovirus), readily trigger attacks of asthma, often followed by a prolonged period of coughing. If you have asthma, it's worth doing all you can to avoid contact with cold sufferers and be ready to double the dose of treatment you're taking to control your symptoms. Like people with allergic rhinitis, you may be one of the one in 20 asthma sufferers who have a severe attack after taking aspirin or other non-steroidal anti-inflammatory drugs such as ibuprofen (Nurofen). Of additional concern to asthma sufferers is the use of tablets used to treat high blood pressure. You should never take one frequently prescribed type of treatment known as the beta-blockers since they block the beneficial effect of the naturally occurring adrenaline in the blood which helps to keep the airways of the lung open. There have been deaths among asthma sufferers who have been prescribed these drugs.

PLANNING
YOUR TREATMENT

The doctors who are managing your asthma will have specific goals in mind when choosing the right treatment for you.

TREATMENT TARGETS

The aims are to ensure that:
- You lead a full active life
- You keep your lung function as near to normal as possible
- You are able to take part in sporting activity if you want to - whether you are an adult or a child
- You lose no time from school or work
- You suffer no night-time symptoms

The emphasis has moved away from treatment of asthma symptoms as they arise and towards giving sufficient anti-allergic and anti-inflammatory treatment to prevent symptoms occurring in the first place. This has led to the development of a step-wise plan (set out on page 38) for the management of asthma with the aim of preventing symptoms and keeping lung function, as measured by the peak flow meter, as near normal as is possible. Should peak flows fall by 20 per per cent from your best recorded measurements, you will need higher doses of anti-allergic and anti-inflammatory treatment. It is vital that you are able to inhale your asthma medications effectively. The advantage of taking medicines in this way is that the amount absorbed into the bloodstream is very low and side-effects are largely avoided.

Spacer devices are helpful for people who find inhalers on their own difficult to use.

It's not always easy to acquire the knack of inhaling the spray from a metered dose inhaler. You have to breathe in whilst at the same time activating the inhaler to release the correct dose. Some people never

THE FIVE TREATMENT STEPS

1 Occasional use of a bronchodilator inhaler, such as salbutamol (Ventolin), terbutaline (Bricanyl). Using this treatment by itself is only recommended if your asthma is very infrequent and your lung function normal.

2 Regular anti-allergic treatment with sodium cromoglycate (Intal), nedocromil sodium (Tilade). This treatment taken regularly is the best therapy if your asthma attacks are occurring on a regular basis and your lung function, as measured by a peak flow meter, is essentially normal.

3 Anti-inflammatory treatment with beclomethasone dipropionate (Becotide), budesonide (Pulmicort) inhalers. These corticosteroid inhalers are extremely effective, when taken regularly, in controlling asthma symptoms and improving lung function, and should be used if anti-allergic treatment is not keeping your asthma under control and your lung function normal. When beclomethasone dipropionate (Becotide) or budesonide (Pulmicort) are used at doses ranging from 100-800 micrograms per day, side-effects are rarely a problem. Occasionally deposition of the aerosol spray at the back of the throat leads to a yeast infection known as candidiasis (thrush). This may cause a sore throat and sometimes weakening of the voice. Brushing your teeth, gargling or eating immediately after using the inhalers is the best way to prevent any of the corticosteroid spray remaining at the back of your throat.

4 High dose anti-inflammatory treatment with budesonide (Pulmicort) at a dose of 1600 micrograms per day, fluticasone propionate (Flixotide), 1-2 mg daily. The use of higher doses of inhaled corticosteroids may be required if your asthma is not controlled using the lower doses or during a bad phase caused, for example, by pollution or the common cold virus. At higher doses these corticosteroids are absorbed into the blood stream to a significant extent and may be associated with some side-effects. Remember to reduce the dose once your symptoms are under control and your lung function improved.

5 Tablets of corticosteroid, prednisolone: This is an emergency treatment for severe attacks of asthma. Tablets of prednisolone taken at high doses above 15 mg/day for long periods of time will

be associated with the development of side-effects. These include indigestion, thinning and bruising of the skin, wasting of muscles, and thinning of the bones. A short course of prednisolone over a few weeks, however, is highly unlikely to be associated with such side-effects and may be necessary to relieve severe symptoms and improve reduced lung function.

manage this technique effectively, but there are many devices available to help. The medicine can be initially sprayed into and then breathed out of a spacer device, so you don't have to synchronise triggering the inhaler and breathing in. Devices which contain the asthma medication in the form of a dry powder are easier to use since after loading the inhaler, all you have to do is simply breathe the powder into your lungs. Such devices include spinhalers, diskhalers and turbohalers. Make sure you use the inhaler device that you find suits you best. As yet none of the medicines needed for the treatment of asthma is available without prescription.

You can use bronchodilator treatment whenever you need it at any step in the treatment of asthma, but remember that if you have to use your inhaler more than four times a day it is best to increase the dose of anti-allergic and anti-inflammatory treatment.

Inhalers are the best way of getting drugs to where they're needed.

Peanut and other food allergies

Reactions to foods are extremely common although only a very small proportion of the symptoms that develop after eating particular foods are true allergies, meaning that they involve the body's immune system. Everyone has their likes and dislikes when it comes to food, and young children often refuse particular foods as part of their drive for independence. However in later life over-eating or rejection of certain foods (food faddism) is usually the result of psychological factors, not clearly understood. The most severe form of food aversion is anorexia nervosa, characterized by a determined refusal to eat which usually begins in adolescence. Anorexics, who can be very manipulative, often persuade their carers that they have severe food allergies causing a wide range of symptoms. In this way they may be able to disguise the anorexia and become classified as suffering from the total allergy syndrome. Apart from aversion, other reactions to foods are best described as food intolerances. Food intolerance encompasses normal reactions to large amounts of specific foods, the irritant effects of foods, results of deficiency in the enzymes necessary to break up foods, and true food allergy.

NORMAL FOOD REACTIONS

Caffeine is the most popular and widely used stimulant drug in the world, and produces side-effects at doses of only 200 mg - just two moderately strong cups of coffee. It is addictive and particularly affects the nerves, the heart and stomach. Too much coffee and your hands shake, your heart races, your oesophagus (food-pipe) relaxes with subsequent heartburn, and your sleep is disturbed. Some cheeses and pickled fish contain tyramine, chocolate contains phenylethylamine, and citrus fruits, octopamine. Bananas, avocados, yeast extract and wine contain similar compounds which can affect and cause widening of the blood vessels, bringing on migraine in susceptible people, flushing of the face and the widespread itchy skin eruption known as nettle rash or urticaria. Histamine is found in some cheeses, sauerkraut, sausages such as pepperoni and salami. Bacteria can produce histamine and high levels of this potent chemical can be found in fish, particularly mackerel if kept too long. Consuming large amounts of histamine causes urticaria, swelling of the lips, face and tongue, and intense headaches.

Some foods can bring on a very unpleasant allergic reaction even in tiny amounts.

IRRITANT EFFECTS

Stomach ache, wind, constipation and diarrhoea are extremely common, affecting almost everyone. The food we eat influences symptoms, altering the tenderness of the gut, production of gas and composition of the faeces - a well-known example being curry powder. The persistence of such symptoms without any serious underlying cause is called the irritable bowel syndrome which is very common and as yet poorly understood. Nevertheless avoiding foods which exacerbate symptoms, increasing the amount of fibre in the diet and learning to cope better with stress, can all be helpful.

ENZYME DEFICIENCY

Low levels of an enzyme called lactase, which breaks down milk, is a rare but important cause of severe watery diarrhoea in children, when they are fed cow's milk. In some ethnic groups, for example the Chinese, where milk plays little part in the diet, levels of lactase are extremely low and drinking milk or eating milk products leads to diarrhoea. Lactase levels may be temporarily reduced by many common bowel disorders such as gastroenteritis and drinking milk can cause diarrhoea for many months following the illness, so it's best to stay off milk until the enzymes return to their normal level. Alcohol is broken down in the body by a series of enzymes, one of which is called aldehyde dehydrogenase. Up to 40 per cent of Japanese people have very low levels of this enzyme and are particularly susceptible to the effects of drinking alcohol, which they learn to avoid.

An enzyme deficiency can prevent some babies from digesting feeds made with cows' milk.

FOOD ALLERGY

Fifteen per cent of the population say that they suffer symptoms related to eating certain foods. It is possible to test this by disguising the food in a specially prepared meal and comparing the effects with the same meal not containing the suspected food allergen. This type of 'blinded food challenge' shows that the true frequency of allergies and intolerances occurs in less than 2 per cent of people. Nevertheless allergy to milk, eggs, fish, and nuts in particular can cause severe symptoms, particularly in children, and allergy to peanuts appears to be increasing at an alarming rate.

The symptoms that develop following contact with a minute amount of the food are well recognized. In highly food-allergic sufferers mere contact between the offending food and the lips causes tingling and rapid swelling of the lips within seconds to minutes. This is followed by swelling of the tongue which if severe enough can cause obstruction at the back of the mouth and suffocation unless the appropriate treatment, in the form of an injection of adrenaline, is rapidly given. If the food has been eaten, the person vomits violently and severely and if some of the food allergen has been absorbed into the bloodstream they develop a widespread urticarial rash, start to wheeze and their blood pressure drops steeply.

This generalized reaction is called anaphylaxis and without treatment can and does lead to tragic loss of life in young people. Sometimes the onset of food allergic symptoms can be more insidious and difficult to diagnose, requiring the expert help of a dietician. The sufferer will be involved in careful research, recording what foods they've eaten over the preceding weeks in a diary which can then be studied in relation to their symptoms.

One of the most difficult problems you'll encounter if you have a food allergy is to know whether prepared foods contain the offending allergen. A good example is peanut allergy.

Peanuts

Fish

Eggs

Milk

Allergy to many foods can cause severe symptoms and allergy to peanuts appears to be increasing at an alarming rate.

One way of confirming the diagnosis is to put the sufferer on a strict elimination diet which includes a very restricted number of foods: for example, one meat, one fruit, one vegetable, one starch source. The choice of foods is based on those least likely to cause allergic reactions, such as lamb or chicken, rhubarb or pears, carrots or sprouts, and rice or potato. A fat source such as a milk-free margarine or specific vegetable oil, and sugar, may also be allowed. If symptoms settle on this strict elimination diet additional foods can then be added and if symptoms develop the source of the problem is easily identified.

Peanut allergy

The peanut (*Arachis hypogea*) is actually related to the pea and is a legume, not a nut. Like other peas it bears its fruit in pods (shells) but the unusual thing is that they develop underground. Between 15-18,000,000 metric tons of peanuts are harvested every year, especially in Asia, Africa and the United States. For anyone who's not allergic to them, they are a very healthy food: there is more protein in peanuts than in the equivalent weight of beefsteak. As well as being a food in itself, the peanut is a greater source of edible oil than almost any other commercially grown crop. Peanuts are passed through rollers which grind them into small particles and then squeezed through a press. Alternatively, a chemical solvent is used to dissolve the oil. It's known that unless specially prepared, peanut oil still contains the peanut allergen, and peanut oil is widely used in prepared foods, both as the oil itself and as a carrier for fat-soluble vitamins and colourings.

Peanuts   Meat

Weight for weight, peanuts contain more protein than steak.

Apart from foods the uses of peanuts are many and various. Low grade oil is used as an ingredient in soaps, shaving creams, shampoos and even paints, and the manufacture of the explosive nitroglycerine. Peanut oil, listed as arachis oil, is a component of some medicinal products including skin care products which might be prescribed for allergic patients. Many children with extreme peanut allergy have never been knowingly exposed to peanuts prior to their first reaction, raising the question of how they became sensitized. Peanut oil was a common constituent of many infant milk formulas, but there is now no peanut oil in Cow & Gate infant milk formulas, Heinz infant milk formula, Milupa, Sainsbury's infant milk formula, or in SMA infant milk formulas. There is still peanut oil in the follow-on milk produced by Boots, but this will be changed. Another concern is that there may be cross-reactivity between peanut and soya, which is a common constituent of infant milk formulas. Research into this is urgently required.

Food additives

A food additive is any substance not commonly used as a food which is added to a food at any stage to affect its keeping quality, texture, consistency, taste or smell. Additives may trigger urticaria, asthma and rhinitis, and the most important colouring causing symptoms is the yellow dye tartrazine (E102), frequently added to many convenience foods. In addition tartrazine is usually present in smoked cod and haddock, lime and lemon squash, salad cream and marzipan, and somewhat surprisingly in mint sauce and jelly, brown sauce and tinned processed peas. Another yellow colouring, sunset yellow (E110), is present in orange squash, fish fingers, lemon curd and Lucozade. Benzoates (E211) are preservatives, preventing the growth of bacteria and fungi and are added to many drinks, for example soft drinks, squashes and beer and also to margarine.

symptoms for you and so avoid consuming them.

DIAGNOSIS

Skin testing and blood tests (RAST and CAP) can be very helpful in identifying food allergy to milk,

THE EUROPEAN FOOD INTOLERANCE DATABANK

It is vital that people suffering from food intolerance and allergy are able to find out what is actually included in various foods. A joint initiative between the British Dietetic Association, the Food and Drink Federation and the Leatherhead Food Research Association led to the development of a database in the UK, and now in Europe, containing details of ingredients and additives. The databank can be accessed by your dietitian. Information from food

retailers and manufacturers is carefully checked and covers the following food additives and ingredients:
Milk, egg, wheat, soya and their derivatives; sulphur dioxide, benzoate, glutamate and azo-colours.
Many supermarket chains now have detailed lists of all the constituents of their prepared foods and some, together with the British Allergy Foundation, have prepared leaflets covering the main food allergies.

The number of people who suffer from reactions to additives is relatively small, possibly a tenth of those who suffer food intolerances. Nevertheless food additives pose a real problem which is being taken increasingly seriously by food manufacturers. Thanks to improvement in labelling it is increasingly possible to identify which foods contain the chemicals that provoke

egg, fish, shellfish, wheat, soya, peanut and true nuts, but blinded food challenges and strict elimination diets may be necessary in the diagnosis of more complex cases.

TREATMENT
Diet

Cutting out the food which is causing your intolerance or allergy is the key to successful treatment.

However, it is vital that you make sure that your diet is nutritionally adequate, providing sufficient protein, energy, vitamins and minerals, particularly calcium. This is especially important in young children whose growth rate can be impaired by poorly designed low-energy elimination diets. Do not adopt a very restrictive diet without professional help from a dietician.

Antihistamines

Antihistamines are useful for the treatment of the milder manifestations of food allergy, where the symptoms are confined to itching and swelling of the lips, swelling of the face (angio-oedema) and urticaria. Loratadine (Clarityn) or cetirizine (Zirtek) are the antihistamines you should opt for. They are, however, of no value in the more severe life-threatening reactions which include swelling of the tongue, asthma, and falling blood pressure.

Epi-pens, Min-i-jets and Medihaler-epi

The only effective treatment for the severe food allergies causing life-threatening reactions is adrenaline. This medicine will cause constriction of the blood vessels in the swollen lips, face and tongue, reverse the asthma, and raise blood pressure. It must be administered rapidly. Swelling within the mouth can be

treated using the Medihaler-epi which is an aerosol of adrenaline: you spray four puffs into your mouth. It is not advisable to use this method of taking adrenaline to deal with more widespread allergic reactions. Treating severe allergic reactions to foods yourself has been revolutionized by the introduction of the Epi-pen auto-injector. This has a spring-activated concealed needle and is designed to deliver a single 0.3 mg dose of adrenaline into a muscle when the pen is pushed firmly against the outer thigh. The children's version contains a dose of 0.15 mg of adrenaline. Min-i-jet adrenaline is an alternative but this consists of a 1 ml disposable syringe and needle, and you have to measure the dose needed since a full syringe will deliver 1 mg of adrenaline. Most people much prefer the Epi-pen which is easy to use, has no needle visible and has a shelf-life of two years compared to the nine months of the Min-i-jet adrenaline.

Adrenaline, delivered through a device called the 'Epi-pen', is used to treat severe allergic reactions.

While the Min-i-jet adrenaline may contain too large a dose of adrenaline the Epi-pen auto-injector may not give a big enough dose to treat severe anaphylactic reactions. For this reason you should always carry two Epi-pens with you, so that you can use the second one 10 minutes after the first if your symptoms are not responding adequately. If you are at risk from severe allergic reactions, you have to get used to carrying the Epi-pens with you wherever you go. When the sufferer is a child, it may be best to have Epi-pens at home and Epi-pens at school. Increasingly, teachers are prepared to administer adrenaline, particularly to use the Epi-pen, once they have had advice and training. Because of the increasing frequency of peanut allergy some schools are becoming nut-free zones.

Medic-Alert and allergy patches

If you have a life-threatening allergy, you must make this fact known so that appropriate treatment can be given if you are unconscious when emergency medical treatment arrives. Medic-Alert provides a bracelet or necklet containing medical details and a 24-hour emergency number. For further details call free on 0800 581420. Allergy patches with the words 'I am allergic to nuts', for example, can be helpful in young children at nursery or primary school.

Fixed on to outer clothing they immediately highlight the sufferer's problem to teachers and other children and parents.

Itchy skin rashes

Raised itchy lumps - urticaria

Urticaria closely resembles the itchy white blisters and red patches that result from nettle stings and the reaction in the skin is mainly due to histamine from mast cells. They can occur on any part of your body, and normally, come and go over the space of a few hours. Acute, short-lasting attacks of urticaria are very common, affecting as many as one in five of the population at some stage in their lives.

Anyone who's allergic to dogs, for example, will rapidly develop a red itchy rash when licked on the face by a dog. Food allergy sufferers frequently develop swelling of the lips or inside of the mouth after eating eggs, milk or nuts. Sometimes this type of contact urticaria can be triggered by intolerances to chemicals including ammonia, bleaches and preservatives, as well as to nettles and the primula plant.

When you eat something you're allergic to, you'll get widespread urticarial rashes all over your body. Well known causes - in addition to milk, egg and nuts - are fish, shellfish, beans, potatoes, strawberries, celery, parsley and spices. You'll get this type of rash following a bee or wasp sting if you're allergic to the venom of these insects, and many medicines, particularly penicillin, are associated with widespread itchy rashes.

If no external cause for the urticaria can be found, and the rash persists over several weeks, then other causes need to be identified. Some people find that changes in

| Before angio-oedema | After angio-oedema |

The skin swelling know as angio-oedema is a reaction to histamine and other chemicals released by mast cells.

temperature and pressure can bring on the rash and in children with this condition a hereditary absence of a blocking protein in the blood may be the cause, particularly if other members of the family are affected. In severe and long-lasting urticaria the body may be reacting against itself with the development of an antibody against the mast cell which causes it to release histamine. You may be one of the many urticaria sufferers who knows the cause of your skin rash so you can avoid the triggering food. In others skin prick testing or RAST may help to discover the offending allergen. Elimination diets may help. Antihistamines are particularly helpful in blocking the effect of histamine

released from mast cells in the skin which causes this itchy rash. Taking a non-sedating antihistamine such as cetirizine or loratadine once a day will relieve the symptoms rapidly and effectively. However, finding a permanent cure means identifying the cause whenever possible and avoiding the allergen once you know what it is.

SKIN SWELLINGS - ANGIO-OEDEMA

Angio-oedema simply means a deep swelling in the tissues, particularly of the face, tongue, and larynx, caused by the effects of histamine and other chemicals released from mast cells which cause the blood vessels to leak fluid

12 months   18 months - 3 years   Over 4 years

Eczema sites alter in a child's first four years of live.

into the tissues. It is closely linked to urticaria with similar causes and like urticaria can be triggered by both allergens and intolerance to a number of medicines as well as preservatives. The commonest triggering factor in up to 75 per cent of sufferers is aspirin and the closely related non-steroidal anti-inflammatory drugs such as ibuprofen (Nurofen). Occasionally paracetamol can be the cause. Preservatives and colourings also need to be avoided, particularly benzoic acid, ascorbic acid, parabens, sulphites and anti-oxidants. One particular type of modern medicine used to treat raised blood pressure and heart failure, known as the angiotensin converting enzyme inhibitors or ACE inhibitors, can cause severe urticaria and angio-oedema. Swelling of the tongue and larynx causes increasing breathlessness and can be fatal unless rapidly treated by injection of adrenaline.

ITCHY CRACKED SKIN

The commonest causes of itchy, scaly, weepy red rash are atopic eczema and contact dermatitis.

Atopic eczema

This rash starts between the ages of two and six months, often on the face, and the irritation keeps the baby awake. The rash can spread over the body but the nappy area is not involved. In about half of the children affected in this way, the rash clears by 18 months of age. In the remainder the rash moves to the skin folds, particularly the inside of the elbows and the backs of the knees. Additionally the skin on the side of the neck, wrists and ankles is affected, and in toddlers eczema often persists on the face.

Atopic eczema is less common in adults. The rash principally affects skin folds where thickening can occur. Emotional problems can prolong the course of the disease but it usually disappears on its own by the age of 30. Localised patches of eczema can occur on the lips and sometimes on the nipples in young women. Eczema may reappear on parts of the body which are under physical stress for some reason - for example, on the hands of nurses and hairdressers. Eczema affecting the hands and feet often appears as small blisters under the skin and in older people patches of eczema are often associated with varicose veins around the ankles.

The part played by allergy to house dust mite, pets, and foods in causing atopic eczema remains controversial. However the National Child Development Study has shown that eczema recorded by physical examination is almost twice as common in better off people as compared to those with lower incomes. This finding indicates that environmental exposure and lifestyle are at least as important as genetic factors in the development of childhood eczema.

Factors which might explain this difference include the amount of carpets and central heating in the home (because of their influence on the house dust mite population), use of showers and soaps, exposure to ultra-violet light, contact with pets, age of the mother and diet. Seventy five per cent of children with severe atopic dermatitis have very high concentrations of IgE antibody to the mite allergen, and patch tests with mite allergens produce a positive result. The application of mite allergen to eczematous skin makes the rash worse and children improve in hospital where mite counts are low, even when they're being given no specific treatment.

Some sufferers notice the development of eczema around their eyes and nose during the pollen season, adding further misery to their allergic conjunctivitis and rhinitis. Twenty five per cent of eczema sufferers are allergic to eggs, milk, nuts, wheat, fish and shellfish. Apart from the development of contact urticaria around the face and mouth on contact with food, sufferers describe itching and worsening of eczema eight to 24 hours later. Eczema often starts after babies are weaned from breast milk and giving them formula milk instead of cows' milk can sometimes cause a dramatic improvement. Similarly, reducing a child's exposure to house dust mite and pets can be helpful. It is possible to at least delay the onset of infant eczema in at-risk babies born to allergic parents by breast feeding as long as possible, avoiding cow's milk, house dust mite control measures, banishing pets and banning smoking in the home.

The basic treatment for eczema is use of emollients and avoiding the use of soap. Sufferers often find that one of the many available emollients suits them better than the others and this should be applied regularly throughout the day and particularly after a bath or shower. If avoiding allergens and using emollients doesn't solve the problem, corticosteroid ointments and creams are the best form of treatment. The key principle is to use the least potent steroid preparation needed to keep eczema under control and when possible stop the treatment for short periods. For many children one per cent cortisone ointment is adequate. Potent steroid creams and ointments should be used with caution for limited periods only.

Some patients have benefited considerably from using evening primrose oil (Epogam) at appropriate doses of 160-320 mg daily in children and 320-480 mg in adults. It's worth trying it for three months if other simpler measures have failed, but if there's no improvement within that time, it's not worth continuing.

CHINESE HERBAL MEDICINE

There are more than 600 clinics offering traditional Chinese medicines which have produced impressive responses in cases of atopic eczema that have proved resistant to conventional medicine. Usually the treatment involves drinking a tea prepared from 10 or so plant materials tailored to the individual patient. Though there is no doubt that some of the plant materials used by the Chinese for treating eczema are beneficial, and in some cases better than Western treatment, the effect unfortunately is usually temporary with a relapse occurring after six to 12 months. In addition the herbal remedies may damage the liver. Careful analysis of the compounds present in the plant materials may in the future lead to better standardized, safer and more effective therapies for eczema.

Antihistamines are of little benefit in the management of atopic eczema. Worsening eczema may be the result of secondary infection with bacteria requiring treatment with the appropriate antibiotic from the doctor.

Allergic contact dermatitis

Unlike allergic eczema this disease is more common with advancing age. Symptoms are redness, scaling and thickening of the skin which itches where it has been in contact with the allergen - for example, on the face with cosmetics and aftershave, and on the ears from the nickel in earrings. The hands are affected in two thirds of contact dermatitis, much of it due to contact with sensitizing agents encountered at work.

Many people with skin conditions find that they're better when they've been out in the sun, but sunlight can itself cause a rash in fair-skinned people. The answer is to use a sun-block cream. Some perfumes, cosmetics, eye lotions and even sunlotions themselves contain chemicals, usually preservatives and antiseptics that make the skin more sensitive to sunlight, as can some antibiotics, leading to a red, itchy rash when you sunbathe.

An increasing and worrying problem is allergy to natural rubber latex used in balloons, condoms and particularly gloves. One in 10 health care workers in the USA are now affected, with the proportion up to 17 per cent in one hospital.

THE COMMON ALLERGENS

Nickel: clothing clasps, spectacle frames, jewellery, coins, household utensils

Chromate: leather, bleaches, matches, cement

Formaldehyde: preservatives, cosmetics, nail varnish, newsprint, cigarettes, fabric conditioners, wrinkle-resistant clothes

Ethylene diamine: preservatives in creams, paints

Mercaptobenzothiazole: rubber products, especially boots, gloves and catheters

Thiurams: rubber products, fungicides in paint and soap

Plants: primula, poison ivy, dahlias and chrysanthemums.

The diagnosis can be confirmed by patch testing and avoiding the allergen is the cure.

The allergy is increasing in Britain as more and more dentists, nurses and health care professionals wear gloves, not just when operating but when taking and handling blood and other bodily fluids.

The reaction varies from allergic contact dermatitis on the hands due to chemicals used in the manufacturing process to urticaria on the hand associated with asthma, anaphylaxis and even death. People with this allergy must ensure that doctors and dentists treating them use non-latex gloves, by wearing a Medic-Alert bracelet or necklet which could be life-saving.

Hypo-allergenic cosmetics

Sixty per cent of women say they have a sensitive skin and hypo-allergenic cosmetics are increasingly popular. Lanolin and particularly preservatives and perfumes are the common skin sensitizers. If you have sensitive or allergy-prone skin, it's best to choose cosmetics without perfume and those containing the minimum of pigments, since each carries its own risk of allergy. Check that products are in narrow-necked tubes or jars since they are less likely to be contaminated with bacteria and preservatives. 'Air-backless' tubes prevent air being sucked in and prevent contamination with bacteria. Don't use products after the expiry date. In 1997 ingredient listing in all cosmetics will become compulsory and sufferers will be able to avoid known sensitizers easily.

Wasp and bee stings

Bees (*Apis mellifera*) and wasps (*Vespula vulgaris*) belong to the Hymenoptera order. Bees are cultivated all over the world for honey and pollination of fruit trees. Hives survive during the winter and you can get stung by a bee on exceptionally warm winter days but it's more likely to happen from spring to autumn. Bumble bees are not very aggressive and stings from them are rare. Wasps have typical black and yellow bodies and wasp waists. They build their nests under ground or in natural or man-made cavities. They live close to humans and are found particularly on over-ripe fruit and sweet foods.

Their aggressive nature makes them the commonest cause of insect sting allergy. Only the queen survives the winter so wasp stings only occur in summer and early autumn. A wasp can withdraw its sting apparatus but a bee loses its stinger which, because of its associated barbs, can work its way deeper into the skin.

The venom contains the allergens mellitin in bees, antigen 5 in wasps, and phospholipase A and hyaluronidase in both. Bee keepers and their families, country dwellers, agricultural workers and keen gardeners are most at risk, but anyone can be stung and allergy can develop just as easily in those who have no other allergies as in those

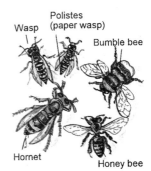

Stings

Wasps are aggressive and more likely to sting you than bees.

who do. Although bee and wasp stings are very common large local reactions at the sting site occur in only 10 per cent of the population with widespread allergic reactions including urticaria, asthma and a falling blood pressure occurring in less than half a per cent. Fortunately deaths are rare in the UK, just five to 10 per year, and even those could be avoided with proper diagnosis and a plan to deal with the emergency.

The diagnosis of wasp and bee sting allergy can be confirmed by skin prick testing or by CAP-RAST, and you should have this done if you ever have a large local skin reaction with redness and swelling extending over 10 cms or any widespread reaction.

TREATMENT

As with all allergies avoidance is the best treatment.

- Don't move suddenly when wasps and bees are around
- Keep away from fallen over-ripe fruit
- Wear gloves when gardening or picking fruit
- Don't wear loose-fitting or brightly coloured clothes
- Don't wear perfume
- Opt out of picnics or alfresco meals
- Never walk barefoot
- Remember that sweat attracts many insects

Emergency treatment

- Remove the sting carefully. Place your nail underneath the venom sac and lift out the sting.
- Large local reactions will respond to an antihistamine such as cetirizine 10 mg (Zirtek) or loratidine 10 mg (Clarityn) and a single dose of prednisolone tablets (50 mg).
- Widespread reactions require emergency treatment with adrenaline.

Use the Epi-pen immediately if you have any difficulty breathing, you feel dizzy or if a rash appears away from the sting. Always carry two Epi-pens wherever you go all year round if you're allergic to bees, and in summer and autumn for wasp allergy.

- Hyposensitization (specific allergen injection immunotherapy). This is the best way to prevent widespread reactions and anaphylaxis to wasp and bee stings. Increasing concentrations and amounts of the venom are injected under the skin (subcutaneously) at weekly intervals for 15 weeks. The top dose, usually 100 micrograms of the venom, is then injected monthly for three years. This provides over 90 per cent protection which lasts for many years. The diagnosis of wasp and bee allergy and hyposensitization treatment can only be provided in specialist hospital centres.

Useful Addresses

The Anaphylaxis Campaign

For information on peanut/food anaphylaxis (that is to say, immediate allergic reaction).
34 George Road
Fleet
Hants GU13 9PS
Tel:(01252) 318723

The British Allergy Foundation (BAF)

This organisation was founded in June 1991 by a group of leading medical specialists determined to improve the awareness, prevention and treatment of allergy. The British Allergy Foundation encompasses all types of allergy and aims to offer information and support to sufferers as well as raising funds for allergy-related research. Work is mainly funded by voluntary income and a small government grant towards the cost of the Allergy Helpline.
St Bartholomew's Hospital
West Smithfield
London EC1A 7BE
Tel: (0171) 600 6127
Allergy Helpline: (0171) 600 6166

The British Lung Foundation

This charity was established in 1985 to raise funds for research into all forms of lung disease. They also have a series of self-help groups around the country, The Breathe Easy Club, which are largely run by patients.
8 Peterborough Mews
Parsons Green
London SW6 3BL
Tel: (0171) 371 7704
Fax:(0171) 371 7705

National Asthma Campaign (NAC)

This is the only charity solely dedicated to asthma. It raises funds for research and is the biggest contributor to asthma research in the UK. It has an active network of local groups run by asthmatics for asthmatics who provide a variety of services to their local population apart from raising remarkable amounts of money for research. It was formed by the amalgamation of the Asthma Society and the Asthma Research Council.
Providence House
Providence Way
Upper Street
Islington, London N1 0NT
Tel: (0171) 226 2260
Asthma Helpline: (0345) 010203

The National Eczema Society

163 Eversholt Street
London NW1 1BU
Tel: (0171) 388 4097

Medic Alert Foundation

For medical SOS necklets & bracelets.
12 Bridge Wharf
156 Caledonian Road
London N1 9UU
Tel: (0171) 833 3034
Freephone: 0800 581420

Ministry of Agriculture, Fisheries & Food

Food Safety Directorate
Chemical Safety of Food Division
For information on all foods.

Room 504A
Eron House
17 Smith Square
London SW1P 3JR
Tel: (0171) 238 6267

J Sainsbury PLC

For information & product guides
on dietary needs.
Stamford House
Stamford Street
London SE1 9LL
Tel: (0171) 921 6000

Index

Understanding

HAY FEVER
& OTHER ALLERGIES

Professor Robert J Davies

CLARITYN & CLARITEYES

Our grateful thanks to Schering-Plough,
makers of Clarityn & Clariteyes, for their
contribution towards the production
of this book

Published by Family Doctor Publications Limited
in association with the British Medical Association

All rights reserved. No part of this publication may be reproduced, or stored in a retrieval system, or transmitted, in any form or by any means, electronic, mechanical, photocopying, recording and/or otherwise, without the prior written permission of the publishers. The right of Professor Robert J. Davies to be identified as the author of this work has been asserted in accordance with the Copyright, Designs and Patents Act 1988 Sections 77 and 78.

IMPORTANT

This book is intended to supplement the advice given to you by your doctor. The author and publisher have taken every care in its preparation. In particular, information about drugs and dosages has been thoroughly checked. However, before taking any medication you are strongly advised to read the product information sheet accompanying it. Your pharmacist will be able to help you with anything you do not understand.

© Family Doctor Publications 1995

Medical Editor: Dr Tony Smith
Consultant Editor: Chris McLaughlin
Front Cover Illustration: Colette Blanchard
Medical Artist: Angela Christie
Design: Fox Design, Bramley, Guildford, Surrey
Printing: Cambus Litho, Scotland, using acid-free paper

ISBN: 1 898205 17 5